I0041651

THE SECRET IN HERBAL MEDICINE

GET RAPID HEALING THROUGH

ALOE VERA PLANT

GINGER PLANT

TURMERIC PLANT

CHAMOMILE PLANT

ECHINACEA PLANT

GARLIC PLANT

"Health is wealth" when you're alive

BY

DR.BEN JAPHETH

TABLE OF CONTENTS:

CHAPTER 1
PLANT USE FOR TREATMENT

CHAPTER 2

CHANGE THAT OCCUR WITHIN THE SYSTEM BETWEEN AGE 20-50, 50-80

CHAPTER 3

HERBAL THAT COULD BOOST YOUR IMMUNE SYSTEM 3.1

INTRODUCTION

The power of herbal drugs has been honored for centuries by numerous societies around the world.
The use of shops and sauces as drugs has been proved throughout history and has been a vital part of traditional drug practices.
Herbal drugs have played an essential part in managing colorful health conditions by offering natural remedies that are accessible, affordable, and, most importantly, effective.
In this essay, I'll bandy the power of herbal drugs and its benefits. Originally, herbal drugs have been preferred over conventional drugs due to their natural origin. utmost conventional drugs are artificial and synthesized in labs, while herbal drugs are deduced from natural sources similar to shops and sauces.
This distinction is vital in the aspect that natural remedies are frequently more permitted by the body than synthetic bones .
The naturally occurring constituents in herbal drugs offer a holistic approach to treating illness, as they work with the body's essential mending capacities.

Unlike numerous conventional specifics, herbal drugs aren't addictive and don't harm the body with long- term use.

Natural remedies give a sustainable volition to precious and frequently dangerous synthetic medicines.

Also, herbal drugs are readily available in numerous corridors of the world and frequently come with minimum costs.

The maturity of medicinal sauces are set up locally, and their medication is frequently straightforward, making them affordable to utmost people.

The commercialization of herbal products might come with significant costs, but the maturity of natural remedies are readily available and fluently accessible.

Due to their low costs, herbal drugs offer an excellent result, particularly in third- world countries where access to healthcare is minimal, and drug costs are generally prohibitive.

A clear illustration of this is the African traditional drug system that's heavily reliant on sauces and has helped millions of people deal with colorful conditions.

In South Africa, herbal drugs are regulated under the Medicines and Related Substances Act, meaning that herbal remedies must undergo the same strict testing as pharmaceutical medicines before they can be sold to the public.

The use of herbal drugs has been successful in treating conditions similar to HIV/ AIDS, tuberculosis, and malaria in Africa.

Likewise, herbal drugs are effective in the operation of habitual conditions similar to diabetes, high blood pressure, and arthritis. Research has shown that colorful sauces have a positive effect on diabetes by regulating blood sugar situations.

Sauces similar to bitter melon, gymnema, and fenugreek have hypoglycemic goods and can help reduce overall blood sugar situations in the body.

Also, colorful sauces similar to garlic, hawthorn berries, and turmeric have shown positive effects on reducing high blood pressure.

In arthritis, herbal remedies have been used to reduce inflammation in the joints. Sauces similar to gusto, boswellia, and turmeric have anti-inflammatory parcels that make them effective in managing arthritis symptoms.

Also, herbal drugs have a significant positive impact on internal health.

For example, sauces similar to passionflower, ashwagandha, and valerian have shown some fantastic results in managing anxiety, depression, and stress.

These sauces have been historically used to calm the mind and help the body relax, perfecting overall well-being.

Also, herbal drugs have many side goods, when compared to numerous conventional specifics, which frequently come with serious side goods.

Side goods of numerous specifics can range from mild to severe, and they can manifest in the gastrointestinal system, cardiovascular system or the nervous system.

Also, numerous specifics can interact negatively with other conventions.

Herbal drugs have only minimal side effects, primarily because the constituents in natural remedies work together with the body's natural processes.
This collaboration produces smaller side goods and is frequently better permitted by cases.
In conclusion, the power of herbal drugs can not be undervalued.

The availability,affordability, and effectiveness of natural remedies make them invaluable in treating colorful conditions.

The significance of maintaining the use of herbal drugs in everyday healthcare practices can not be ignored.

Ongoing exploration and testing can develop new and advanced herbal treatments that can address more complex health issues.
It's time for the world to embrace herbal drugs as a natural and effective volition to conventional drugs.

HISTORICAL USES OF HERBAL MEDICINE

Historical Use of Herbal

For centuries, humans have reckoned on the mending power of nature to treat colorful affections. The use of sauces as drugs is a practice that dates back to ancient times. Literal substantiation suggests that our ancestors used shops and sauces to cure conditions and promote heartiness. Although ultramodern drugs have replaced numerous traditional remedies, herbal drugs still play a vital part in the health and heartiness assiduity. This essay will explore the literal use of sauces and their significance in ultramodern times. Sauces have been used for medicinal purposes since ancient times. Ancient societies similar to the Greeks, Romans, and Egyptians considered sauces to be a precious resource for maintaining health and precluding illness. The Greek croaker

Hippocrates, who's known as the father of ultramodern drugs, recommended the use of sauces to cure conditions. He believed that nature handed everything that humans demanded to maintain good health. One of his notorious quotations states," Let food be thy drug and drug be thy food." This quotation highlights the belief that food, sauces, and other natural coffers can cure and help conditions.

In ancient Egypt, records indicate that shops were used to treat multitudinous affections similar as constipation, indigestion, and infections. Papyrus calligraphies from 1550 BCE describe the use of sauces similar to aloe vera and frankincense to treat different conditions. Also, the Indian Ayurvedic system of drugs relies heavily on the use of sauces. The system dates back over 5000 times, and its interpreters believe that sauces can profit specific body types and promote health and heartiness. Medieval times were also a significant period for the use of sauces in drugs.

During the medieval period, preachers, monks, and nuns were frequently the sole keepers of knowledge, including medical knowledge.

These religious numbers were responsible for treating the sick, and they reckoned on sauces and other natural coffers for mending. This period saw the arrival of condiment auditoriums , where these religious numbers grew medicinal sauces for use in treating the ill. Sauces have played a pivotal part in Western drug's development, with numerous sauces serving as the base for ultramodern specifics. shops similar asSt. John's Wort, which has been used for centuries to treat depression, is now constantly used for the same purpose.

The natural anodyne morphine is deduced from opium poppies, while aspirin was first created in the late 1800s from willow dinghy. In recent times, the use of sauces and natural remedies has gained fashionability among individualities seeking a more holistic approach to healthcare. Herbal drug is a form of reciprocal and indispensable drug(CAM) that has been gaining interest in ultramodern times.

CAM refers to any practice that isn't part of conventional drugs. As the name suggests, CAM treatments are used alongside conventional drugs to promote and maintain heartiness.

This approach is grounded on treating the body as a whole rather than just fastening on symptoms of an illness. One significant advantage of herbal drugs is its low cost, making it accessible to numerous people who can not go to conventional drugs.

   Herbal drug has been used for different affections similar as anxiety, depression, digestive issues, respiratory infections, and skin issues.

For illustration, gusto is known for its anti-inflammatory parcels, which makes it useful in treating numerous health conditions similar to arthritis and migraines.

Also, chamomile is extensively used for its comforting parcels to treat anxiety and promote relaxation. Echinacea is known for its vulnerable- boosting parcels, making it useful in treating snap and flu.

In conclusion, the use of sauces as drugs is a practice that has been employed for centuries across different societies and societies.

Ancient societies similar to the Greeks, Romans, Egyptians, and Indians all honored the mending power of sauces, which they used to treat affections.

The Middle periods saw the blossoming of condiment auditoriums , where religious numbers grew medicinal sauces for use in treating the sick. In ultramodern times, the use of sauces, and CAM in general, is growing in fashionability. The advantages of herbal drugs include its low cost, availability, and its focus on treating the body as a whole.

While numerous traditional remedies have been replaced with ultramodern drugs, the literal use of sauces and their significance in ultramodern times can't be overlooked.

Chapter 1

PLANTS USE FOR TREATMENT

Shops have been used for medicinal purposes for thousands of times, with early records dating back to ancient societies similar as the Egyptians and Chinese. With the development of ultramodern drugs in recent centuries, the use of factory- grounded treatments has declined; still, numerous people still turn to natural remedies for colorful affections. In this essay, we will bandy colorful shops used for treatment and their medicinal parcels.

ALOE VERA PLANT

Aloe vera belongs to the family of Xanthorrhoeaceae. It has been used for medicinal purposes for centuries in different corridor of the world, especially in Asia, Africa, and Latin America. Aloe vera is known for its remedial parcels that make it precious in treating a variety of health issues. In this essay, we will explore the colorful uses of Aloe vera in health, beauty, and husbandry. One of the most significant operations of Aloe vera is its use in the treatment of skin and hair problems.

Aloe vera gel has a high attention to polysaccharides and glycoproteins that offer a defensive and hydrating effect on the skin. The gel contains an array of vitamins, minerals, and antioxidants, videlicet Vitamin E, Vitamin C, zinc, and selenium, which are known to enhance the skin's vitality. Aloe vera also has anti-inflammatory parcels that soothe the skin and minimize greenishness and lump. According to a study published in the Journal of Bangladesh Society of Physiologists in 2018, Aloe vera gel had significant benefits in treating acne vulgaris and precluding the development of scars. Also, Aloe vera is largely effective in relieving sunburns and nonentity mouthfuls due to its anti-inflammatory and antiseptic exertion. The factory contains composites like aloin and emodin, which reduce pain, itching, and inflammation associated with sunburns and nonentity mouthfuls. therefore, it's used in numerous creams, poultices, and ointments for the treatment of becks

and skin vexations. In addition to skin benefits, Aloe vera is extensively used to promote hair health. The factory's juice is rich in enzymes that are effective in removing dead skin cells and redundant oil painting, which can help unclog hair follicles and encourage hair growth. It also contains Vitamins A, C, and E, which are known to nourish the crown and hair follicles. A study published in the Journal of Chemical and Pharmaceutical Research suggested that Aloe vera gel could also help hair loss and promote hair regrowth in individualities with androgenetic alopecia(manly pattern baldness). piecemeal from health and beauty benefits, Aloe vera has significant operations in husbandry. The factory is known for its failure- resistant parcels, which make it valuable in thirsty and semi-arid regions. It requires little water and can survive in poor soils with low nutrient content. Aloe vera can be grown in glasshouses

or fields and can be gathered several times a time. The factory's gel and juice contain factory growth hormones like auxins and gibberellins, which are known to enhance the growth and yield of crops. A study published in the Journal of Agricultural and Food Chemistry in 2012 stated that applying Aloe vera gel to tomato shops increased their growth rate and fruit yield significantly. In conclusion, Aloe vera is an incredibly protean factory that offers multitudinous health, beauty, and agrarian benefits.

It's extensively used in the ornamental and pharmaceutical diligence to develop natural and effective skin and hair care products. Also, it has a precious part in husbandry as a failure-tolerant and nutrient-rich crop that can enhance crop yields. further studies are demanded to explore the full eventuality of Aloe vera and its different operations completely.

Still, its remedial parcels shouldn't be overlooked, and Aloe vera should be considered as one of the most precious natural remedies available to us.

One of the most extensively known shops used for medicinal purposes is aloe vera. Aloe vera is a succulent factory that's native to northern Africa and has been used for its mending parcels for thousands of times. It's generally used to treat becks
, cuts, and other skin vexations due to its anti-inflammatory and antibacterial parcels. Aloe vera contains a substance called mucopolysaccharides, which helps to stimulate the vulnerable system and promote mending.
Also, aloe vera is rich in antioxidants that help to cover against free revolutionaries and reduce inflammation.

STEPS TO PREPARE ALOE VERA MEDICINE

Aloe vera has been used over centuries for its medicinal parcels. moment, it's extensively used in the pharmaceutical assiduity in the product of drugs, cosmetics, and salutary supplements.
Indeed, aloe vera is incredibly protean, and there are multitudinous ways to prepare it for medicinal purposes. In this essay, we explore how to prepare aloe vera

drugs. Old leaves from the aloe vera factory contain the loftiest medicinal parcels, making them ideal for medications.

Harvest the leaves by cutting them near the base of the factory with a sharp cutter, taking care not to damage the factory. Collect a sufficient number of leaves in a handbasket.

STEP 1

The first step in preparing the aloe vera is to clean the leaves. wash them completely under cold water to remove dirt, bugs, and other pollutants. Pat them dry with a kerchief, and also trim off the saw-toothed edges of the leaves and discard them. Remove the skin of each splint by running a sharp cutter along the edges of the splint to produce a fat, flat subcaste. Set the skin away for composting.

Way 2 Next, separate the gel from the aloe vera pulp by running the cutter blade along the aloe vera's meat to detach it from the rind. Gently remove the gel to help it from breaking into small pieces. Collect the gel in a coliseum, rather made of wood, plastic, or glass, since essence can reply with the gel. Aloe vera gel has an emotional range of remedial parcels.

It possesses anti-inflammatory, antioxidant, and antibacterial parcels, which help in treating numerous affections.

For topical medications, aloe vera gel works well as a skin moisturizer, while internally, it's recommended as a digestive aid. We now explore some ways of preparing aloe vera for_specific medicinal purposes.

PREPARATION IN TERM OF MOISTURE

To prepare an aloe vera gel for a moisturizer, mix the aloe vera gel with avocado oil painting, rose oil painting, and many drops of vitamin E oil painting.
The avocado oil painting nourishes the skin, while rose oil painting provides an affable aroma. Vitamin E is added for its antioxidant parcels, enhancing the moisturizing effect of the aloe vera gel. Stir the constituents well and pour the performing admixture into a glass jar. Apply the gel to the asked area of your skin and rub it gently until absorbed. This admixture can be stored in the fridge for over a week.

PREPARATION IN TERMS OF DIGESTION

Aloe vera can also help palliate digestive issues. Crush one teaspoon of aloe vera gel along with a piece of gusto in a mortar and pestle to form a paste. Add the paste to a glass of warm water and stir well. gusto aids in the digestion process by reducing bloating and gas. Drink the admixture before reflections. This medication will help boost your digestion, easing symptoms like constipation, stomach ulcers, and acid reflux.

PREPARATION FOR BURN

In cases of becks
For sunburns, aloe vera is effective in furnishing a cooling and soothing effect.
To prepare an aloe vera gel for becks
,mix the aloe gel with many drops of coconut oil painting and lavender oil painting to form a paste. Apply the paste on the affected area of the skin and let it dry. Lavender oil painting has anti-inflammatory and pain-relieving parcels, making it a great natural remedy for becks.
Coconut oil painting helps in nourishing the skin, while its antimicrobial parcels help infections.
This admixture can be stored in the fridge in a watertight vessel for over two weeks. In conclusion, aloe vera gel has multiple remedial uses. Proper medication styles

are vital to maximize its medicinal benefits. For topical operations, it's vital to mix it with other suitable constituents depending on the intended use. While for internal operations, it's essential to consult a croaker to help determine the applicable cure grounded on an existent's age, health status, and intended effect.

CHAMOMILE

Another factory generally used for treatment is chamomile. Chamomile is a condiment that's native to Europe, but can now be set up throughout the world. It's generally used in teas and other herbal remedies to help with anxiety, wakefulness, and digestive issues. Chamomile contains a substance called apigenin, which acts as an opiate and helps to promote relaxation and sleep. Also, chamomile has anti-inflammatory parcels that can help to reduce pain and inflammation in the body.

Chamomile Herbal and its Side Effects

Chamomile has been used as a herbal drug for centuries, with its origins tracing back to ancient Egypt, Greece and Rome. Its remedial benefits have been honored by numerous societies around the world. Chamomile flower is used for making herbal tea, essential canvases and other herbal medications. It's believed to have colorful health benefits like relieving anxiety, treating wakefulness, and reducing inflammation. Still, like other herbal drugs, chamomile also has side goods that druggies should be apprehensive of. This essay aims to bandy the implicit side goods of chamomile and how they can affect the stoner's health. One of the enterprises associated with chamomile is that it can beget antipathetic responses in some people. Indeed though the prevalence of similar responses is rare, they can be severe and indeed life-hanging in some cases.

Chamomile can beget antipathetic responses analogous to other shops in the daisy family, like feverfew and ragweed. Thus, people who are apathetic to these shops might also be antipathetic to chamomile. Antipathetic responses can manifest as skin rashes, hives, or itching. In severe cases, it can beget anaphylaxis, a life-hanging condition characterized by swelling of the throat and difficulty in breathing. Another implicit side effect of chamomile is its impact on blood sugar situations.

Chamomile is known to have glucose- lowering goods, which can be salutary for people with diabetes. Still, it can also beget hypoglycemia, a condition characterized by low blood sugar situations. Hypoglycemia can beget symptoms like dizziness, confusion, sweating, and indeed loss of knowledge if left undressed. Thus, people with diabetes who are taking specifics to control their blood sugar situations should cover their glucose situations regularly while using chamomile. They should also consult their medical guru before adding chamomile to their diurnal routine.

Chamomile can also interact with certain specifics, which can beget adverse goods. For illustration, chamomile can increase the goods of opiate specifics like benzodiazepines, barbiturates, and some antidepressants.

This can beget inordinate dizziness, dizziness, and confusion. Chamomile can also interact with anticoagulants like warfarin, causing their goods to be enhanced. This can increase the threat of bleeding, which can be dangerous, particularly for aged grown-ups. piecemeal from these side goods, chamomile can also beget side goods analogous to other herbal drugs.

These side goods include dizziness, fatigue, headache, and gastrointestinal disturbances like nausea, puking, and diarrhea.

These side goods are generally mild and go down on their own after a short while. In conclusion, chamomile is a herbal drug with multitudinous implicit health benefits.

Still, it's essential to be apprehensive of its implicit side effects. Antipathetic responses, hypoglycemia, and drug relations are some of the side goods of chamomile.

Thus, people who are using chamomile should consult with their healthcare provider before using chamomile. They should also be apprehensive of its implicit side goods and cover their symptoms precisely. By following these preventives, druggies can enjoy the benefits of chamomile without passing any adverse side goods.

STEPS TO PREPARE CHAMOMILE MEDICINE

Step 1 Harvesting Chamomile

The first step in preparing chamomile drugs is to gather the chamomile. Chamomile is a flowering factory that belongs to the daisy family. It's stylish to gather chamomile in the morning when the flowers are completely open and have just started to wilt. The flowers are also plucked from the stems and collected in a handbasket.

Step 2 Drying Chamomile

The coming step is to dry the chamomile. Drying chamomile is essential to save its medicinal parcels and help it from spoiling. There are colorful ways to dry chamomile, including air drying, sun- drying, and oven drying.

Air drying is the most traditional system of drying chamomile. It involves spreading the flowers in a single subcaste on a clean and dry face and allowing them to dry naturally over many days.

Sun-drying involves spreading the flowers on a clean face and placing them in direct sun for many hours every day until they're fully dry. Roaster drying involves placing the flowers on a baking distance and drying them at a low temperature in the roaster for many hours.

Step 3 Grinding Chamomile

Once the chamomile has dried, the coming step is to grind it into a fine greasepaint. Grinding chamomile helps to save its medicinal parcels and makes it easier to use in different forms of drug, similar to tea or a tinge. A coffee grinder or a mortar and pestle can be used to grind the chamomile into a fine greasepaint.

Step 4 Making Chamomile

Tea Chamomile tea is a popular form of chamomile drug. To make chamomile tea, boil water in a tea kettle or a pot. Add one teaspoon of chamomile greasepaint for every mug of water. Let the admixture steep for five twinkles before straining it into a mug. Chamomile tea can be candied with honey or sugar and served hot or cold.

Step 5 Making a Chamomile tinge

A chamomile tinge is another form of chamomile drug. To make a chamomile tinge, fill a glass jar with dried chamomile flowers and cover them with vodka or another high- evidence alcohol. The rate of chamomile to alcohol should be one part chamomile to two corridor alcohol. Seal the jar and let it sit in a cool and dark place for two to six weeks, shaking it daily. After two to six weeks, strain the tinge into a clean jar or bottle. For lozenge, it's stylish to consult with a healthcare professional.

In conclusion, chamomile drugs can be set fluently in the comfort of your home. By following the simple way outlined in this essay, you can gather, dry, grind, and use chamomile in different forms of drug, similar to tea or a tinge. Chamomile has been used for centuries for its comforting and soothing parcels, and these ways will help you make the utmost of this condiment.

GINGER PLANT

Gusto is another factory that's frequently used for medicinal purposes. gusto is a root that's generally used in Asian cookery, but it also has a long history of use as a natural remedy. gusto is known for its capability to soothe nausea and vomiting, making it an effective remedy for morning sickness and stir sickness. It also has anti-inflammatory parcels that can help to reduce pain and inflammation in the body.

POSITIVE AND NEGATIVE EFFECTS OF GINGER

POSITIVE EFFECTS

Gusto, also called Zingiber officinale, is a root condiment used for medical and culinary purposes for centuries. It's known for its racy and pungent taste and is generally used as a seasoning agent in food and potables.
Gusto contains colorful antioxidant and anti-inflammatory composites that offer several health benefits. The purpose of this essay is to explore the

positive goods of gusto on overall health and good. Originally, gusto has been shown to reduce pain and inflammation.

Gusto contains composites similar to gingerols, shogaols, and parasols that have potent anti-inflammatory parcels. These composites help to reduce inflammation in the body, which can beget habitual pain, similar as arthritis, by blocking prostaglandins' product. A study published in the Journal of Medicinal Food set up that taking 2 grams of gusto per day for 11 days reduced muscle pain by 25 in people performing elbow exercises compared to the placebo group. We can also use gusto for reducing menstrual pain as shown in studies conducted on women passing pain. Cases who consumed gusto daily had a significant reduction in menstrual pain intensity when compared to cases who took a placebo. Hence, gusto's anti-inflammatory parcels make it a natural and effective anodyne, without the negative side goods generally associated with specifics.

Secondly, gusto aids in digestion and helps help nausea. gusto is also used as a digestive aid and is specified as a home remedy for digestive diseases like indigestion, flatulence, and dyspepsia. Its digestive parcels help bloating and gas conformation, leading to proper digestion. gusto has been shown to increase digestive enzymes, thereby abetting in digestion.

Also, gusto contains composites that help reduce nausea and puking associated with gestation, chemotherapy, and surgery.

A review published in the Journal of Ethnopharmacology suggested that gusto may help reduce the inflexibility of nausea and puking in cancer cases witnessing chemotherapy. Therefore, gusto is a natural and safe result for digestive issues and nausea.

Thirdly, gusto contributes to heart health in colorful ways. A study conducted on cases with heart complaint showed that taking gusto supplements lowered triglyceride situations, which are fats set up in the blood. High situations of triglycerides can lead to heart conditions. Another study published in the International Journal of Cardiology set up that gusto supplementation can help reduce the threat of diabetes and the associated cardiovascular conditions.

Also, gusto consumption has also been set up to help drop blood pressure in hypertensive cases. Hence, gusto's donation to heart health is essential, and incorporating it into one's diet can help reduce the threat of heart conditions.

Fourthly, gusto helps promote healthy brain function.
A study published in the substantiation- Grounded reciprocal and Indispensable Medicine journal suggested that gusto's antioxidant parcels cover the brain from oxidative stress and inflammation. Oxidative stress and inflammation are linked to neurodegenerative conditions like Alzheimer's complaint and Parkinson's complaint.

Likewise, gusto consumption has been set up to help ameliorate cognitive function and memory in healthy middle-aged women. Hence, gusto is an excellent

addition to a healthy diet as it supports brain health and function. In conclusion, gusto is a salutary root condiment that offers several health benefits. gusto has anti-inflammatory parcels, which make it effective in reducing pain, similar to menstrual cramps. gusto also aids in digestion, which promotes healthy gut and bowel chronicity. Also, gusto helps promote heart health by lowering triglyceride situations and reducing blood pressure in hypertensive cases. gusto promotes healthy brain function by furnishing antioxidants that cover the brain from oxidative stress and inflammation. These positive goods of gusto make it a natural volition to conventional specifics while furnishing an effective and safe result for colorful health issues.
Citations - Black CD, Herring MP, Hurley DJ,O'Connor PJ. J Med Food. 2010; 13(5) 679- 83. doi 10.1089/ jmf.2009.1374. PMID 20418184.

NEGATIVE EFFECTS

Gusto, a root belonging to the Zingiberaceae family, is an extensively used component in colorful cookeries and artistic practices. It's also well- known for its medicinal parcels and has been traditionally used to treat digestive and respiratory diseases, inflammation, and pain. Still, despite its multitudinous benefits, gusto also has negative goods that need to be taken into consideration.

One of the primary negative goods of gusto is its capability to beget stomach worries and vexation. gusto has been known to increase the product of stomach acid, which can lead to nausea, bloating, and indeed heartburn. This effect is particularly pronounced in individuals with preexisting gastrointestinal conditions similar as peptic ulcers, gastroesophageal reflux complaint(GERD), and seditious bowel complaint(IBD). For these individualities, the consumption of gusto can complicate their symptoms and beget further discomfort. Another negative effect of gusto is its eventuality to interact with certain specifics. gusto can enhance the goods of blood-thinning specifics similar as warfarin and aspirin, which can increase the threat of bleeding.

It can also interact with specifics used to lower blood sugar situations, similar as metformin and insulin, leading to hypoglycemia. Also, gusto can intrude with blood pressure specifics and beget an unforeseen drop in blood pressure, leading to dizziness and fainting. Likewise, gusto has been linked to antipathetic responses in individuals who are sensitive to it. An antipathetic response to gusto can present with symptoms similar to skin rash, itching, blown lips or lingo, and difficulty breathing. These symptoms can be severe and bear immediate medical attention.

In addition to the forenamed negative goods, inordinate consumption of gusto can also lead to other adverse goods similar as diarrhea, indigestion, and mouth vexation. gusto, when taken in large quantities, can also lead to a drop in platelet aggregation and increase the threat of bleeding. This effect can be dangerous for individualities witnessing surgery or those with bleeding diseases.

In conclusion, gusto has several positive health benefits, but its negative effects can not be ignored. gusto can beget stomach worries, interact with certain specifics, beget antipathetic responses, and lead to several other adverse goods.

Thus, it's essential to consume gusto in temperance and to consult a healthcare provider before using it as a treatment for any health condition.

HOW TO PREPARE GINGER MEDICINE

Gusto is a popular root used in traditional drugs. It has been used for medicinal purposes for centuries because of its remedial parcels. gusto is abundant in gingerols, which are phenolic composites that give gusto its characteristic taste and scent. gusto can be prepared in a variety of ways for medicinal purposes, similar as tea, greasepaint, saccharinity, and capsules. In this essay, we will be agitating on ways to prepare gusto drugs.

1. Choose fresh gusto root

The ideal selection for making gusto drug is fresh gusto root. Fresh gusto gives the stylish result for gusto drug but if unapproachable, dried gusto could be used rather. Make sure to choose indefectible and knotty gusto as those are the freshest.

2. Clean the gusto root

Gusto root must be gutted duly before use. The root must be washed completely using an encounter to remove any dirt or contaminations. wash the gusto well under running water to remove any remaining debris.

3. Peel the gusto root

Peel off the external subcaste of the gusto root as it can be tough to bite , hard to digest, and adds a woody flavor. Using the aft end of a ladle can help scrape off the skin without wasting any gusto meat.

4. **Gusto is a popular**

 root used in traditional drugs. It has been used for medicinal purposes for centuries because of its remedial parcels. gusto is abundant in gingerols, which are phenolic composites that give gusto its characteristic taste and scent. gusto can be prepared in a variety of ways for medicinal purposes, similar as tea, greasepaint, saccharinity, and capsules. In this essay, we will be agitating on how to prepare gusto drugs.

PROCESS FOR PREPARING GUSTO DRUG

•Choose fresh gusto root- The ideal selection for making gusto drug is fresh gusto root. Fresh gusto gives the stylish result for gusto drug but if unapproachable, dried gusto could be used rather. Make sure to choose indefectible and knotty gusto as those are the freshest.

•Clean the gusto root- gusto root must be gutted duly before use. The root must be washed completely using an encounter to remove any dirt or contaminations. wash the gusto well under running water to remove any remaining debris.

•Peel the gusto root- Peel off the external subcaste of the gusto root as it can be tough to bite , hard to digest, and adds a woody flavor. Using the aft end of a ladle can help scrape off the skin without wasting any gusto meat.

•Cut the gusto- Cut the gusto into thin slices or small pieces for use in the drug- making process. The thing is to cut the gusto into small enough pieces that it'll release its essential canvases during the birth process.

• Boil the gusto- Add the gusto pieces to a saucepan of water and heat. Bring it to a pustule and let it poach over low heat for 10- 15 twinkles. This process releases the gingerols, and the longer the boiling time, the stronger the gusto flavor will come. Once coddled, turn off the heat and let it cool.

• Strain the gusto water- After the boiling process, strain the gusto water using a fine- mesh strainer or cheesecloth. The solids can be discarded, and the liquid can be used as a base for gusto tea, saccharinity, or other medicinal medications.

• Saccharinity Making To make a gusto saccharinity, blend equal corridors of gusto water and honey or sugar. Store in a jar and chill for over 1 month. One teaspoon of saccharinity in warm water can be taken for a cough, sore throat, or digestive issues.

• Ginger Capsules For gusto capsules,

 mix one part of dried gusto greasepaint with two corridors of a neutral flour- suchlike rice flour, mix well. Fill empty capsules using a capsule filling machine. Preparing gusto drug at home is an affordable and natural way of treating affections that bear gusto's medicinal parcels. gusto is useful for nausea, puking, indigestion, cold wave, cough, and indeed headaches. Making gusto drugs can be an easy process that can be done using simple kitchen implements. The benefits of gusto drugs are innumerous, and it's an effective way to relieve several symptoms. In conclusion, gusto drugs can be prepared by following simple ways similar to choosing fresh gusto, cleaning, shelling, boiling, straining, making saccharinity, or preparing capsules. Making gusto drugs is an excellent volition to using over-the-counter specifics with adverse side goods. By making and consuming manual gusto drugs, we can ameliorate and maintain our health effectively.

Cut the gusto into thin slices or small pieces for use in the drug- making process. The thing is to cut the gusto into small enough pieces that it'll release its essential canvases during the birth process.

5. **Boil the gusto**

Add the gusto pieces to a saucepan of water and heat. Bring it to a pustule and let it poach over low heat for 10-15 twinkles. This process releases the gingerols, and the longer the boiling time, the stronger the gusto flavor will come. Once coddled, turn off the heat and let it cool.

6. **Strain the gusto water**

- After the boiling process, strain the gusto water using a fine- mesh strainer or cheesecloth. The solids can be discarded, and the liquid can be used as a base for gusto tea, saccharinity, or other medicinal medications.

7) **Saccharinity Making**

To make a gusto saccharinity, blend equal corridors of gusto water and honey or sugar. Store in a jar and chill for over 1 month. One teaspoon of saccharinity in warm water can be taken for a cough, sore throat, or digestive issues.

8) **Ginger Capsules**

For gusto capsules, mix one part of dried gusto greasepaint with two corridors of a neutral flour- suchlike rice flour, mix well. Fill empty capsules using a capsule filling machine.

Preparing gusto drug at home is an affordable and natural way of treating affections that bear gusto's medicinal parcels. gusto is useful for nausea, puking, indigestion, cold wave, cough, and indeed headaches. Making gusto drugs can be an easy process that can be done using simple kitchen implements.

The benefits of gusto drugs are innumerous, and it's an effective way to relieve several symptoms. In conclusion, gusto drugs can be prepared by following simple ways similar to choosing fresh gusto, cleaning, shelling, boiling, straining, making saccharinity, or preparing capsules. Making gusto drugs is an excellent volition to using over-the-counter specifics with adverse side goods.

By making and consuming manual gusto drugs, we can ameliorate and maintain our health effectively.

TURMERIC PLANT

Turmeric is a spice that's generally used in Indian cookery, but it's also used for its medicinal parcels.Turmeric contains a substance called curcumin, which has important anti-inflammatory and antioxidant parcels.

It has been shown to help with a wide range of health issues, including arthritis, heart complaint, and cancer. Also, curcumin has been shown to ameliorate brain function and reduce the threat of Alzheimer's.

POSITIVE AND NEGATIVE EFFECTS OF TURMERIC

POSITIVE EFFECTS

Turmeric, the bright unheroic spice generally set up in Indian and Middle Eastern dishes, has been used for centuries as a natural remedy for a variety of health conditions. The active element of turmeric, curcumin, is an antioxidant and anti-inflammatory agent that has been linked to multitudinous positive health goods. In this essay, we will explore some of the positive goods of turmeric on the body. One of the most well- known benefits of consuming turmeric is its anti-inflammatory parcels. Inflammation is a natural response of the vulnerable system to heal the body from injury or infection.

Still, habitual inflammation has been linked to multitudinous habitual conditions similar to heart complaint, diabetes, and cancer.

Curcumin has been shown to suppress certain motes in the body that are responsible for inflammation, making it an important tool in precluding and managing habitual complaints. Another positive effect of turmeric is its capability to support brain health.

Curcumin has been set up to increase situations of a hormone called Brain- deduced Neurotrophic Factor(BDNF).

BDNF is responsible for the growth and survival of neurons, which are essential for cognitive function. Low situations of BDNF have been linked to conditions similar as Alzheimer's and depression. By adding BDNF situations, turmeric has the implicit to ameliorate brain function and cover against these conditions. Turmeric has also been set up to be salutary for cardiovascular health.

One study set up that curcumin supplementation significantly reduced cholesterol situations in fat individuals with high cholesterol.

High situations of cholesterol can lead to the buildup of shrines in the highways, which can ultimately beget heart complaints.

By reducing cholesterol, turmeric may help heart complaints.

In addition to promoting heart health, turmeric has also been linked to a lower threat of developing certain types of cancer.

Various research is proven that curcumin can inhibit the growth and spread of cancer cells .

One study set up that curcumin was effective in reducing the number of colon cancer cells in a laboratory setting.

While further exploration is demanded to completely understand the implicit cancer-fighting benefits of turmeric, these primary findings are promising.

One of the lower-known benefits of turmeric is its eventuality to ameliorate skin health. Turmeric has been used for centuries in Ayurvedic drugs as a treatment for colorful skin conditions, including psoriasis and eczema. The Anti-inflammatory parcels of curcumin may help reduce greenishness and inflammation associated with these conditions.

Also, turmeric has been set up to have antibacterial parcels, which may help acne and other bacterial skin infections. Away from its positive goods on physical health, turmeric may also have benefits for internal health. One small study set up that curcumin was effective in reducing symptoms of anxiety in individuals with a generalized anxiety complaint.

While further exploration is demanded in this area, these primary findings suggest that turmeric may be implicit as a natural treatment for anxiety.

Overall, the positive goods of turmeric on the body are multitudinous and varied.

From reducing inflammation and supporting heart health to potentially precluding cancer and perfecting skin and internal health, there are numerous reasons to add this important spice to your diet. Whether consumed in supplement form or added to reflections, turmeric is an easy and succulent way to boost your health and good. . 2009; 41(1) 40- 59. - Demesne KS.

goods of Curcumin in Inflammatory Conditions of the Gastrointestinal Tract and the Central Nervous System. Libraries of Pharmacal Research. 2021; 44(2) 169- 180.

NEGATIVE EFFECTS

As one of the most common spices in the world, turmeric has been known as a natural remedy for colorful conditions. Turmeric, also known as Curcuma longa, is a root that has been used in Ayurvedic drug for over 4,000 times. It contains an active emulsion called curcumin, which has potent antioxidant and anti-inflammatory parcels. While the benefits of turmeric are extensively accepted, not numerous people are apprehensive of its implicit negative side goods. In this essay, we will explore the negative goods of turmeric on the mortal body. One of the most current negative goods of turmeric is its impact on the digestive system.

While the spice has been used to treat digestive issues in history, it can beget stomach worries, nausea, and diarrhea in some individuals. According to a study published in the Journal of Medicinal Food, taking large boluses of curcumin can lead to gastrointestinal problems similar to diarrhea and nausea. The study set up that taking a high cure of turmeric on an empty stomach can beget stomach vexation and discomfort in some individuals. Likewise, turmeric can negatively impact individualities with gallbladder problems.

Gallbladder problems are common, with roughly 10-15 of grown-ups suffering from gallstones, inflammation of the gallbladder, or other gallbladder issues.

According to a report published in the World Journal of Gastroenterology, turmeric has been shown to increase the product of corrosiveness, which is stored in the gallbladder. This can beget the gallbladder to contract, leading to discomfort or pain for those with gallbladder issues. Another negative effect of turmeric is its impact on blood clotting.

Turmeric has been shown to have antiplatelet parcels, which means it can intrude with blood clotting. This can be salutary for those at threat of blood clots or who have had a heart attack, as it can help further clotting. Still, for those who are formerly taking blood thinners or have a bleeding complaint, the use of turmeric can increase the threat of bleeding and bruising.

A study published in the Journal of Clinical & Diagnostic Research set up that turmeric can affect the body's clotting process, and those taking blood-thinning specifics should consult with their croaker

before taking turmeric supplements. In addition to the impact on the digestive system and blood clotting, turmeric can also negatively affect manly fertility. According to a study published in the Journal of supported Reproduction and Genetics, men who consumed turmeric on a frequent basis had dropped sperm attention and motility. The study set up that turmeric had a negative effect on the morphology and function of sperm, which can contribute to manly gravidity. While the study was conducted in vitro, the experimenters suggest that men trying to conceive should avoid consuming large quantities of turmeric. In conclusion, while turmeric has been shown to have multitudinous health benefits, it's essential to be apprehensive of the implicit negative side effects. Turmeric can beget stomach worries, nausea, and diarrhea, particularly when taken in large boluses on an empty stomach. It can also lead to discomfort or pain for those with gallbladder issues, affect the body's clotting process, and drop manly fertility.However, it's pivotal to consult with your croaker

to ensure it's safe for you and your specific health requirements, If you're taking turmeric supplements or considering using turmeric for its health benefits.

STEPS TO PREPARE TURMERIC MEDICINE

Turmeric has been used in traditional drugs for centuries, and with further exploration being conducted on its health benefits, it's getting increasingly popular as a natural remedy for a range of conditions. Turmeric is a factory that belongs to the gusto family, and it's the root of the factory that's used to make drug. The active component in turmeric is called curcumin, which is a potent antioxidant and anti-inflammatory. In this essay, we will discuss the way to prepare turmeric drugs.

These ways will help you to make a potent and effective turmeric remedy that you can use to help with a variety of health conditions.

Step 1 Choose the Right Turmeric

The first step to making turmeric drugs is to choose the right turmeric. You want to look for turmeric that's fresh and of high quality. You can find fresh turmeric root in utmost health food stores or online. It's important to note that turmeric root can be relatively delicate to find in some areas, so you may need to search for a original or online store that stocks it. When you're opting turmeric, it's important to look for organic turmeric. This is because non-organic turmeric may contain dangerous chemicals or fungicides that can be dangerous to your health. You should also look for turmeric that's rich in curcumin, as this is the active component that provides the health benefits.

Step 2 Wash and Prepare the Turmeric

Once you have named your turmeric, the coming step is to wash and prepare it. You should first wash the turmeric completely to remove any dirt or debris on the face. You can use a vegetable encounter to drop the turmeric root gently to remove any remaining patches. After the turmeric is clean, you can begin to prepare it for consumption. There are a many different ways to do this, depending on the type of drug you want to make. One simple way is to grate the turmeric and mix it with hot water to make a tea. Alternatively, you can blend the turmeric with other constituents similar to honey, gusto, or bomb to make a more potent remedy.

Step 3 Cook the Turmeric

Once you have prepared your turmeric, the coming step is to cook it. This is important because cooking the turmeric releases the active component curcumin, making it more potent and effective.

There are many different styles for cooking turmeric, depending on the type of drug you want to make. One popular way to cook turmeric is to poach it in water or milk for several twinkles. This creates a turmeric paste that you can also use in a variety of different remedies. Alternatively, you can add the turmeric to a saucepan with other spices and constituents similar to ghee, black pepper, and cinnamon to make a more complex remedy.

Step 4 Store the Turmeric Medicine

Once you have cooked your turmeric, the final step is to store it duly. Turmeric remedies can be stored in many different ways, depending on the type of drug you have made.

Still, you can store it in a watertight vessel in the refrigerator for over two weeks, If you have made a turmeric paste. Alternately, you can indurate the paste for longer storage.However, you can either store it in the refrigerator or indurate it in ice cell servers for a longer storehouse, If you have made a turmeric tea.

Conclusion Turmeric is an important and protean medicinal factory that has been used for centuries. By following the way outlined in this essay, you can make your own effective and potent turmeric remedies at home. Flashback to choose high- quality, organic turmeric, marshland and prepare it precisely, cook it duly to release the active component curcumin, and store it rightly for optimal energy. With these ways in mind, you can start to enjoy the numerous health benefits of this amazing factory.

ECHINACEA PLANT

Echinacea is a condiment that's generally used for its vulnerable- boosting parcels. It's native to North America and has been used by Native American lines for centuries. Echinacea is generally used to help and treat the common cold wave and other respiratory infections. It contains composites that help to boost the vulnerable system and reduce inflammation in the body. These are just a many examples of shops used for medicinal purposes. As you can see, there are numerous different shops that have unique parcels and can be used to treat a wide range of health issues. While ultramodern drug has clearly revolutionized healthcare, it's important to flash back that there are still numerous natural remedies that can be effective and safe. In conclusion, shops have been used for medicinal purposes for thousands of times and continue to be used moment.
Aloe vera, chamomile, gusto, turmeric, and echinacea are just a many examples of shops used for treatment. Each of these shops has unique parcels that can help to promote mending and ameliorate overall health. While it's important to consult with a healthcare professional before starting any new treatment, natural remedies can be a safe and effective option for numerous people.

POSITIVE AND NEGATIVE EFFECTS OF ECHINACEA PLANT

POSITIVE EFFECTS

Echinacea is a factory that has been employed for its medicinal parcels for centuries. It has been traditionally used as a herbal remedy to boost the vulnerable system and promote mending. The factory is native to North America and was originally used by the indigenous peoples for its health benefits. Echinacea is presently a popular component in numerous untoward supplements, teas, and creams. This essay explores some positive goods of Echinacea on mortal health backed by scientific and anecdotal substantiation. Echinacea has been set up to have a positive effect on the mortal vulnerable system. According to exploration, Echinacea stimulates the vulnerable system by adding leukocyte exertion, which in turn can increase the body's capability to repel viral, bacterial, and fungal infections. A study conducted in 2015 by Sharma et al. set up that the consumption of Echinacea increased the product of several vulnerable system labels, including white blood cells and natural killer cells, which are essential for fighting off infections. Another study by Percival et al. set up that individuals who took Echinacea supplements endured smaller cases of respiratory infections than those who did not. These findings suggest that Echinacea has a potent immunomodulatory effect. Also, Echinacea has been set up to have anti-inflammatory parcels that can be useful in treating colorful medical conditions. Inflammation is a process by which the vulnerable system responds to infections or injuries, and inordinate inflammation can have negative counter accusations for overall health. A review of several studies conducted by Anheyer et al. in 2018 set up that Echinacea can reduce inflammation in the body by dwindling the situations of seditious labels like C-reactive protein. This Anti-inflammatory effect has been observed to profit individuals with rheumatoid arthritis and other seditious conditions. Echinacea may also have an impact on internal health. Stress is a common factor that negatively affects internal health. individuals who are constantly exposed to stressors may witness habitual inflammation, wakefulness, and anxiety. According to a study conducted by Jawna- Zboinska etal. in 2018, Echinacea excerpt can initiate a stress response that improves the body's adaptability to stress. In the study, actors who were given Echinacea were set up to have lower situations of cortisol, a hormone that's frequently elevated during stressful situations. The study concluded that Echinacea excerpt may be a useful natural remedy for individualities who witness habitual stress. Likewise, Echinacea has been set up to be a natural remedy for skin cells that are growing. One study by Newall et al. set up Echinacea to have antioxidant exertion that can help neutralize free revolutionaries, which contribute to cellular damage and skin aging. The study further asserts that Echinacea can ameliorate the skin's appearance by reducing wrinkle conformation and adding humidity retention. In conclusion, Echinacea has multitudinous benefits for mortal health. It has vulnerable- boosting parcels,anti-inflammatory goods, a positive influence on internal health, and can act as a natural remedy for growing skin cells.

While numerous of these parcels are supported by anecdotal substantiation, scientific studies give compelling substantiation for the use of Echinacea as a natural supplement to ameliorate overall health. With its expansive pharmacological benefits, Echinacea provides a feasible volition to pharmaceutical curatives for individuals who are seeking natural and effective remedies for their health conditions. Citations Sharma,M., Anderson,M., Schoop,R., & Hudson,J.B.(2015). Antiviral exploration, 123, 113- 119.

NEGATIVE EFFECTS

Echinacea is a popular factory- grounded supplement that's extensively used for its purported health benefits, particularly for enhancing the body's vulnerable system. Echinacea is frequently retailed as a" natural" remedy for everything from the common cold wave to infections and other affections. Still, while echinacea has some implicit remedial goods, it's also associated with a range of negative side goods and implicit pitfalls that druggies should be apprehensive of.

In this essay, we will explore some of the negative goods of echinacea. originally, it's important to fete that while echinacea is frequently touted as a important vulnerable- system supporter, there's actually veritably little dependable substantiation to support numerous of its claims. While some early studies suggested that echinacea could be effective in reducing the inflexibility and duration of the common cold wave, more recent exploration has failed to confirm these findings. In fact, a comprehensive review of the being exploration on echinacea and the common cold wave concluded that" the substantiation for the efficacy of echinacea in the treatment or forestallment of the common cold wave is weak and inconsistent"(Barrett et al., 1999).

Secondly, echinacea has been associated with a range of negative side goods and implicit health pitfalls. One of the most generally reported side goods of echinacea is gastrointestinal torture, including nausea, puking, diarrhea, and stomach cramps.

Other implicit side goods include dizziness, headaches, and antipathetic responses. Also, some studies have suggested that echinacea may intrude with certain specifics, particularly medicines used to treat autoimmune conditions.

This is because echinacea can stimulate the vulnerable system, which may complicate autoimmune symptoms or intrude with the effectiveness of specifics(McKenna et al., 2002). Likewise, there's veritably little standardization or regulation of echinacea product and use, which means that it can be delicate to determine exactly what you're getting when you use echinacea supplements.

Different echinacea shops can vary significantly in the situations and types of active composites they contain, and numerous echinacea supplements may be defiled with other substances. This lack of standardization and regulation make it delicate to estimate the safety or implicit pitfalls of using echinacea. In conclusion, while echinacea is frequently seen as a natural and inoffensive supplement, it's important for druggies to be apprehensive of its implicit negative goods and pitfalls.

There's limited scientific substantiation to support numerous of the claims made about echinacea's effectiveness, and there's substantiation to suggest that it can beget a range of negative side goods and indeed intrude with certain specifics. Also, the lack of standardization and regulation of echinacea product and use leaves implicit druggies in the dark about the composition and implicit pitfalls of the supplements they're taking.

Given these enterprises, it's important to approach echinacea with caution and to consult with a healthcare professional before taking any supplements or specifics.

STEPS TO PREPARE ECHINACEA MEDICINE

Echinacea is a popular factory- grounded supplement that's extensively used for its purported health benefits, particularly for enhancing the body's vulnerable system. Echinacea is frequently retailed as a" natural" remedy for everything from the common cold wave to infections and other affections. still, while echinacea has some implicit remedial goods, it's also associated with a range of negative side goods and implicit pitfalls that druggies should be apprehensive of. In this essay, we will explore some of the negative goods of echinacea. originally, it's important to fete that while echinacea is frequently touted as a important vulnerable- system supporter, there's actually veritably little dependable substantiation to support numerous of its claims. While some early studies suggested that echinacea could be effective in reducing the inflexibility and duration of the common cold wave, more recent exploration has failed to confirm these findings. In fact, a comprehensive review of the being exploration on echinacea and the common cold wave concluded that" the substantiation for the efficacity of echinacea in the treatment or forestallment of the common cold wave is weak and inconsistent"(Barrett etal., 1999). Secondly, echinacea has been associated with a range of negative side goods and implicit health pitfalls. One of the most generally reported side goods of echinacea is gastrointestinal torture, including nausea, puking, diarrhea, and stomach cramps.

Other implicit side goods include dizziness, headaches, and antipathetic responses. Also, some studies have suggested that echinacea may intrude with certain specifics, particularly medicines used to treat autoimmune conditions. This is because echinacea can stimulate the vulnerable system, which may complicate autoimmune symptoms or intrude with the effectiveness of specifics(McKenna et al., 2002). likewise, there's veritably little standardization or regulation of echinacea product and use, which means that it can be delicate to determine exactly what you're getting when you use echinacea supplements.

Different echinacea shops can vary significantly in the situations and types of active composites they contain, and numerous echinacea supplements may be defiled with other substances.

This lack of standardization and regulation make it delicate to estimate the safety or implicit pitfalls of using echinacea.

In conclusion, while echinacea is frequently seen as a natural and inoffensive supplement, it's important for druggies to be apprehensive of its implicit negative goods and pitfalls.

There's limited scientific substantiation to support numerous of the claims made about echinacea's effectiveness, and there's substantiation to suggest that it can beget a range of negative side goods and indeed intrude with certain specifics. Also, the lack of standardization and regulation of echinacea product and use leaves implicit druggies in the dark about the composition and implicit pitfalls of the supplements they're taking. Given these enterprises, it's important to approach echinacea with caution and to consult with a healthcare professional before taking any supplements or specifics

GARLIC PLANT

Garlic is a largely nutritional factory that has been used for thousands of times in colorful societies as a food and drug. It's part of the Allium family, along with onions, shallots, and leeks, and is known for its pungent odor and characteristic taste. In this essay, we will discuss the history, civilization, and health benefits of garlic. Its use was wide in ancient Egypt, Greece, and Rome, where it was valued for its medicinal parcels. In ancient Rome, garlic was used to treat a variety of affections, including digestive problems, respiratory diseases, and high blood pressure. It was also believed to ward off evil spirits and was used in religious observances. At the moment, garlic is most generally used as a culinary component, adding flavor to a variety of dishes. It's also extensively used in supplements and herbal remedies for its implicit health benefits. Garlic is an imperishable factory that's easy to grow and can be cultivated in utmost climates. It's generally grown from cloves, which are individual units that make up the garlic bulb. These cloves are planted in the fall and gathered in the late spring or early summer. There are two main kinds of garlic: hardneck and softneck. Hardneck garlic is known for its larger cloves, which are easier to peel, while softneck garlic has lower cloves. Hardneck kinds also produce a central stalk, or elude, which can be gathered and used in cuisine. Garlic requires well- drained soil and plenty of sun to grow. It's generally planted in rows and should be fertilized regularly to ensure healthy growth. When the garlic bulbs are ready to be gathered, they should be dug up and allowed to dry in a warm, dry place for several weeks. One of the most well- known health benefits of garlic is its eventuality to lower cholesterol and reduce the threat of heart complaint. Garlic contains composites called allicin and alliin, which have been shown to reduce cholesterol situations and ameliorate blood inflow. In addition, garlic has been shown to have anti-inflammatory parcels, which can help to reduce the threat of habitual conditions similar to arthritis and cancer. Garlic has also been shown to have antibacterial and antiviral parcels, which can help to boost the vulnerable system and fight off infections. In one study, garlic was set up to be effective against a variety of bacteria, includingE. coli and salmonella. In addition to its implicit health benefits, garlic is also a great source of nutrients. It's high in vitamin C, vitamin B6, and manganese, and is also a good source of fiber. While garlic is generally considered safe for utmost people, there are some preventives that should be taken. Garlic can interact with certain specifics, including blood- thinning specifics and some antibiotics. It may also beget stomach worries and bad breath in some individuals.

In conclusion, garlic is a protean and nutritional factory that has been valued since ancient times for its medicinal parcels. It's easy to grow and can be used in a variety of dishes or taken as a supplement to promote health and heartiness.

While further exploration is demanded to completely understand the benefits of garlic, it's clear that this pungent condiment has a lot to offer.

POSITIVE EFFECTS OF GARLIC

Garlic, a culinary chef, native to Central Asia, is a popular component in numerous dishes around the world. It isn't only succulent, but garlic has been credited with multitudinous health benefits over the times. Then are some positive goods of garlic that make it an essential addition to our diet. Originally, garlic is known to have anti-inflammatory parcels. Inflammation is the body's response to injury or infection and is a vital part of the mending process. still, habitual inflammation can beget numerous health problems like heart complaint, cancer, and Alzheimer's. Studies have suggested that consuming garlic can help combat inflammation in the body. According to a study published in the Journal of Immunology Research," garlic excerpt has the power to reduce inflammation in the body by regulating cytokine product and therefore, can help the onset of habitual seditious conditions"(Tingshu, Wang, Xue, Wu, Liu, &

Xia, 2019). thus, incorporating garlic into our diet can be salutary in precluding the onset of seditious conditions. Secondly, garlic has been linked with maintaining a healthy heart. Heart complaint is one of the leading causes of death worldwide, and multitudinous factors can lead to heart complaint.

High blood pressure, cholesterol, and triglyceride situations are some of the most significant pointers of heart complaint.

Garlic has been shown to have a positive effect on these factors. According to a study published in Lipids in Health and Disease," Garlic can lower blood pressure, drop total cholesterol, and triglyceride situations"(Ashraf, Asghar, Shabbir, & Sultan, 2005). The study also set up that garlic can reduce the threat of developing shrine buildup in the highways, which can contribute to heart complaint. It's essential to note that although garlic has been shown to have a positive effect on the heart, incorporating garlic alone into our diet may not be enough to help heart complaint. A balanced diet and healthy life are essential for heart health. Thirdly, garlic is honored for its antibacterial and antiviral parcels. Garlic has been used to fight infections for hundreds of times. Allicin, an emulsion set up in garlic, has potent antibacterial and antiviral parcels. According to a study published in Food Science and Human Wellness," garlic has broad-diapason antimicrobial exertion against colorful bacterial and viral pathogens"(Chang, Tsai, Lai, Hsieh, & Wang, 2014). These parcels can help fight against infections caused by bacteria and contagions, like the common cold wave. Garlic also has antioxidant parcels that help to cover the body from oxidative damage. Oxidative damage is one of the leading causes of aging and numerous conditions like cancer, Alzheimer's, and Parkinson's. Antioxidants serve to neutralize dangerous free revolutionaries, which beget oxidative damage.

NEGATIVE EFFECTS OF GARLIC

Garlic is a factory that has been used for medicinal purposes for centuries. It has been touted for its numerous health benefits, including its capability to lower blood pressure, boost the vulnerable system, and indeed fight cancer. Still, despite these benefits, there are also some negative effects of garlic that shouldn't be ignored. One of the most common negative goods of garlic is its strong odor. Garlic contains an emulsion called allicin, which is responsible for its pungent odor. This odor can be delicate to get relieve of, and it can be a major turnoff for some people. In addition, the odor of garlic can loiter on the breath for hours after it has been consumed, making it delicate to fraternize or indeed have a discussion with others. Another negative effect of garlic is its eventuality to beget digestive issues. Garlic contains fructans, which is a type of carbohydrate that can be delicate for some people to digest. These fructans can beget bloating, gas, and other digestive discomfort in some people, especially if consumed in large quantities. Also, garlic can interact with certain specifics, including blood thinners. Garlic acts as a natural blood thinner, which can increase the threat of bleeding in individualities who are taking blood thinning specifics. In addition, garlic may also interact with specifics used to treat HIV/ AIDS, so it's important for people who are taking these specifics to talk to their healthcare provider before consuming garlic. Another implicit negative effect of garlic is its capability to beget skin vexation. Some people may develop a rash or other skin vexation when they come into contact with garlic. This is known as garlic dermatitis and is more common in people who are sensitive to the factory. Eventually, some people may be antipathetic to garlic. Garlic dish inclinations are rare, but they can be serious. Symptoms of a garlic mislike may include hives, difficulty breathing, and indeed anaphylaxis. People who suspect they may be antipathetic to garlic should avoid consuming it and talk to their healthcare provider. In conclusion, while garlic has numerous health benefits, it's important to be apprehensive of its implicit negative goods. Garlic can beget digestive issues, skin vexation, and interact with certain specifics. In addition, its strong odor can be a major turnoff for some people. Still, as with any food or supplement, it's important to listen to your body and talk to your healthcare provider if you have any enterprises.

Citations - Borlinghaus,J., Albrecht,F., Gruhlke,M.C.H., Nwachukwu,I.D., & Slusarenko,A.J.(2014). Allicin chemistry and natural parcels. motes(Basel, Switzerland), 19(8), 12591 – 12618. https//doi.org/10.3390/molecules190812591- Zeng,T., & Zhang,C.L.(2016). Garlic and gastric cancer A critical review. Journal of Nutrition and Metabolism, 2016, 3014769. https//doi.org/10.1155/2016/3014769

STEPS TO PREPARE GARLIC MEDICINE

Garlic, also known as the" stinking rose", has been used for colorful health benefits for centuries. It's a part of the onion family and contains essential nutrients that have antimicrobial and anti-inflammatory parcels. One of the significant uses of garlic is in the medication of garlic drug. Below are the ways involved in preparing garlic drugs.

Step 1 Collecting the garlic

The first and foremost step in preparing garlic drugs is collecting the garlic. Garlic can be fluently set up in any grocery store or request. still, one should make sure to buy fresh garlic and not the dried one. The quality and type of garlic one uses have a significant impact on the effectiveness of the drug.

Step 2 Peeling and crushing the garlic

 Once the garlic is collected, the coming step is to peel and crush them. Shelling garlic can be a grueling task as its skin tends to stick to the cloves. One can use a cutter or buy a garlic bobby
to make this task easier. It's essential to crush the garlic as it helps in releasing the enzymes. Crushing also

improves the bioavailability of the active constituents of garlic.

Step 3 Choosing the right detergent

After crushing the garlic, the coming step is to choose the right detergent. The choice of solvent depends on the intended use of the garlic drug. Water is the most generally used detergent, but other detergents like ginger and oil painting can also be used. The detergent must be of good quality and free from contaminants.

Step 4 Soaking the garlic

The coming step is to soak the crushed garlic in the chosen detergent. The duration of soaking varies depending on the type of detergent used and the intended use of the drug. For illustration, if water is used as a detergent, soaking it for many hours would be sufficient. Still, if ginger is used, soaking it for a week may be necessary.

Step 5 Straining the garlic

After soaking, the garlic must be strained to separate the liquid from the solid residue. One can use a strainer or a cheesecloth to strain the garlic. The simulated liquid is the garlic drug, and one can discard the solid residue.

Step 6 Storing the garlic drug

After straining, the garlic drug must be stored in a clean and watertight vessel. It's essential to label the vessel with the name of the drug, the date of medication, and the intended use to ensure that the drug is used mostly. Garlic drugs have several health benefits and can be used for colorful purposes. It's known to reduce the threat of cardiovascular conditions, lower blood pressure, and ameliorate cholesterol situations.

Garlic also has antimicrobial parcels and has been used for treating respiratory infections, sore throats, and observance infections. In conclusion, preparing garlic drug involves six significant ways, videlicet collecting garlic, shelling and crushing garlic, choosing the right detergent, soaking garlic, straining garlic, and storing garlic drug. It's essential to follow these way precisely to ensure that the garlic drug is of good quality and effective. Garlic drugs have been used for centuries as a natural remedy for colorful health issues, and with the below way, one can fluently prepare it at home.

CHAPTER 2

CHANGE THAT OCCUR WITHIN AGE 20-50 IN THE SYSTEM

As we progress, our bodies suffer colorful changes, and our health status is no exception. From age 20 to 50, significant changes take place in our bodies, impacting our physical and internal health. In our 20s, we're at the peak of our physical health. Our bodies are at their height, and we've the energy to do whatever we want without significant limitations. Still, we shouldn't take our health for granted during this time and engage in healthy habits to maintain our well- being. Regular exercise, a balanced diet, and a healthy sleep authority are essential habits to cultivate during our 20s. Engaging in these conditioning can lead to enhanced muscle strength and better cardiovascular health. Also, our vulnerable system is robust at this age, and we've a lower threat of developing numerous conditions. Still, as we approach our 30s, the metabolism slows down, leading to gradual weight gain.

Also, our muscle mass starts to drop, and our bones become weaker, leading to increased chances of developing osteoporosis. We need to be more conservative about our diet and exercise authority during this stage of our lives. Proper nutrition, weight-bearing exercises, and calcium supplements can help maintain our bone viscosity and strength. As we progress, our bodies face an increased threat of developing habitual conditions like high blood pressure, heart complaint, and cancer.

Still, visionary measures can help, detain, or alleviate these issues. For example, we can reduce our threat of heart complaints by quitting smoking, maintaining healthy blood pressure situations, and engaging in regular physical exertion.

Salutary changes like incorporating further fruits, vegetables, and whole grains can also contribute to lower threat situations.

Also, early discovery and treatment of health issues can help reduce their impacts on our lives. Mental health is also a pivotal aspect of our overall health. As we progress, our threat of developing depression, anxiety, and other internal health enterprises increases.

It's important to prioritize internal health by rehearsing tone-care, seeking remedy when necessary, and creating healthy managing mechanisms. Engaging in physical exertion, sharing in social conditioning, and planning are some proven strategies to enhance internal health.

In conclusion, our health status undergoes significant changes between age 20 to 50. The transition from our 20s to our 30s marks a significant shift in our physical health. While we've further energy and abundance in our 20s, dwindling metabolism and muscle mass loss are some of the challenges we face in our 30s. As we progress, the threat of developing habitual conditions and internal health conditions increases.

Nonetheless, visionary measures like healthy life habits, regular check- ups, and early discovery and treatment of health issues can minimize the pitfalls associated with aging.

CHANGE THAT OCCUR WITHIN AGE 50-80 IN THE SYSTEM

As we progress, changes do within the body's systems, leading to changes in functionality and geste
. These changes can happen at any point in life, but they come more pronounced as we reach age 50 and further. In this essay, we will examine some of the changes that occur in the body's systems between the periods of 50 and 80. One of the most significant changes that do as we age is a drop in muscle mass and strength.

This is caused by a drop in the product of mortal growth hormone and testosterone.

As a result, senior individuals may witness dropped mobility and lesser difficulty completing diurnal conditioning similar as climbing stairs or performing ménage chores. Also, bone viscosity decreases with age, leading to an increased threat of fractures and falls. Exercise and strength training can neutralize these goods to some extent. Another change that occurs in the body as we age is a decline in the effectiveness of the vulnerable system. This decline is due to a reduction in the product of T-cells and other vulnerable cells. As a result, senior individualities may witness further frequent infections and ails, as well as dropped response to vaccinations. It's essential to maintain good health habits, similar to frequent handwashing, regular exercise, and sufficient sleep to strengthen the vulnerable system. The cardiovascular system also undergoes changes as we progress, including an increased threat of hypertension and atherosclerosis. High blood pressure can lead to an increased threat of heart complaint, stroke, and order failure. Atherosclerosis, or the buildup of adipose deposits in the highways leading to the heart and brain, can beget casket pain and increase the threat of heart attack or stroke. espousing a healthy life, including exercise and a healthy diet, can help combat these conditions. The digestive system is also affected by growing, leading to constipation and an increased threat of colon cancer. As we progress, the muscles in the digestive tract come less effective, leading to dropped motility and the need for further fiber in the diet.

Also, infections and other ails can lead to dropped appetite and weight loss.However, seek medical advice, If you witness patient digestive issues. The nervous system also undergoes changes as we progress. sensitive capability, similar to hail and vision, may drop, leading to dropped capability to communicate with others.

Also, cognitive function may drop, leading to memory loss, difficulty with problem-working, and dropped capability to learn new information. Engaging in mentally stimulating conditioning, similar to reading and mystifications, can help maintain cognitive function. In conclusion, as we progress, changes within the body's systems lead to differences in functionality and geste.

These changes are the result of a combination of genetics and environmental factors, similar to diet and life choices. Despite these changes, it's possible to maintain good health and functionality through a combination of exercise, healthy eating, and other life habits. It's essential for senior individualities to stay informed about these changes, and seek medical advice when necessary to maintain optimal health and function.

CHAPTER 3

HERBAL THAT COULD BOOST YOUR IMMUNE SYSTEM

Sauces have been used for medicinal purposes for centuries. numerous of them contain parcels that could boost our vulnerable systems naturally. Given the current health extremity, it's essential to explore natural remedies to strengthen our impunity.

One of the most well-known sauces that have been used for vulnerable system support is Echinacea. Echinacea is a part of the daisy family, and it's generally set up in North America. The roots, leaves, and flowers of the factory are used to make drugs to treat colorful nails, including the common cold wave and the flu. Echinacea contains active substances that could strengthen our vulnerable systems by enhancing our vulnerable cell's exertion.

Studies have shown that Echinacea has antimicrobial goods and could reduce the duration of upper respiratory tract infections. Another condiment that could boost our vulnerable system is Elderberry.

Elderberries are dark grandiloquent berries that come from the European Elder tree, which is native to the corridor of Europe and North Africa. Elderberries have been used in traditional medicine for centuries because of their vulnerable system- boosting parcels and high situations of antioxidants. Elderberries contain composites called anthocyanins, which could help our vulnerable system fight off contagions. According to a study published in the Journal of International Medical Research, elderberries could dock the duration and inflexibility of the flu. While sauces could boost our vulnerable systems, it's important to note that they aren't a cover for medical treatment. These sauces could be used as a supplement to our health authority to strengthen our vulnerable systems. It's also essential to consult with a healthcare professional before taking herbal supplements, especially if you have a beginning health condition or take drugs. piecemeal from Echinacea and Elderberry, other sauces and supplements that could boost our vulnerable systems include garlic, gusto, ginseng, and VitaminC. Garlic contains an emulsion called Allicin, which could help our vulnerable system fight contagions and bacteria. gusto contains Gingerols, which could reduce inflammation and boost our vulnerable systems. Ginseng has been shown to enhance the exertion of vulnerable cells and increase our resistance to ails. Vitamin C is an important antioxidant that could cover our vulnerable cells from damage and support the product of white blood cells that fight off infections. In conclusion, sauces have been used for medicinal purposes for centuries. Echinacea and Elderberry are just two of the sauces that could boost our vulnerable systems naturally. While these sauces could be used as a supplement to our health authority, it's important to consult with a healthcare professional before taking any supplements, especially if you have a beginning health condition or take drugs.

It's imperative to concentrate on having a healthy and balanced life to strengthen our vulnerable systems.

This includes eating a healthy and balanced diet, getting enough sleep, managing stress, and regularly exercising. Citations -F. Shah,M.A. Tariq,S.D.N. Nazir,H.M.B. Khan(2019) Echinacea species A medicinal factory with multiple pharmacological and remedial operations, Current Pharmaceutical Design, 25(34), 3654- 3674. https//doi.org/10.2174/1381612825666191118153900-A. Tiralongo &S. Wee(2016) Leucid ®(excerpt of Echinacea purpurea condiment) for precluding and treating the common cold wave, The Cochrane Database of Methodical Reviews, 2016(8), CD013638. https//doi.org/10.1002/14651858.CD013638

CHAPTER 4

FOOD AND NUTRIENTS FOR AGE 50-80

As people age, their nutritive conditions change, and it's important to maintain a healthy diet to stay healthy and active. According to a report by the World Health Organization, good nutrition for aged grown-ups can help habitual conditions, reduce the threat of functional decline, and ameliorate cognitive function. In this essay, we will explore the significance of food for people between the periods of 50- 80. One of the primary enterprises for aged people is maintaining a healthy weight. As metabolism slows down with age, it's important to control calorie input and consume the right proportion of macronutrients. The American Heart Association recommends a balanced diet consisting of whole grains, spare proteins, and healthy fats. Similar foods can help maintain a healthy weight, help heart complaints, and lower the threat of type 2 diabetes.

Foods grandly in fiber are particularly important for aged grown-ups as they prop digestion and help constipation. Whole grains, fruits, and vegetables are excellent sources of salutary fiber. It's also important to consume enough calcium and vitamin D to maintain bone health. Dairy products similar to milk, rubbish, and yogurt are good sources of calcium, while sun and fortified foods contain vitaminD.

Another pivotal aspect of nutrition for aged grown-ups is hydration. As people age, the sensation of thirst diminishes, and dehumidification can lead to serious health issues. Drinking plenitude of water and fluids similar to tea, coffee(decaf), and fruit authorities can help maintain hydration situations.

It's also essential to consume antioxidants to help age-related conditions. Berries, nuts, and lush flora are rich in antioxidants and can cover against oxidative stress caused by free revolutionaries. Omega-3 adipose acids set up in fish similar as salmon and sardines are also critical for maintaining a healthy brain, reducing inflammation, and precluding heart complaints. Consuming a variety of foods is pivotal for a balanced diet. Aged grown-ups may be more prone to salutary scarcities due to a drop in appetite or a limited range of food choices. Thus, they should incorporate a variety of fruits and vegetables of different colors, spare proteins, whole grains, and healthy fats in their diet to meet their nutrition conditions. In addition to the physical health benefits, a balanced and healthy diet can also ameliorate internal health and cognitive function.

Studies have linked a Mediterranean- style diet(rich in fruits, vegetables, whole grains, and healthy fats) to lower rates of depression and anxiety in aged grown-ups.

The nutrients in healthy foods can also ameliorate cognition, memory, and attention span, reducing the threat of madness and cognitive decline. In conclusion, proper nutrition is pivotal for aged grown-ups to maintain their overall health and well- being.

A balanced diet consisting of whole grains, spare proteins, fruits, vegetables, and healthy fats can help help habitual conditions, maintain a healthy weight, and ameliorate internal health. Acceptable hydration, consumption of antioxidants, and a variety of foods are also pivotal for a healthy diet. As we progress, our nutritive conditions change, and it's essential to acclimatize and maintain a healthy diet to stay healthy and active.

CHAPTER 5

THINGS TO AVOID AT AGE 50-80

As we progress, it becomes more important to take care of our bodies and minds. There are certain effects that we should avoid doing in order to maintain our health and well-being. Then there are some effects to avoid at age 50- 80.

1. Smoking is one of the worst effects that you can have for your health.
It increases your threat for cancer, heart complaints, stroke, and other serious conditions.However, it's no way too late to quit, If you bomb.

2.Drinking too much alcohol inordinate alcohol consumption can damage your liver, increase your threat for certain types of cancer, and beget other health problems.However, it's stylish to do so in temperance, If you choose to drink.

3. Poor diet Eating a diet rich in fruits, vegetables, whole grains, and spare proteins can help you maintain a healthy weight and reduce your threat for habitual conditions. Avoid reused foods, sticky drinks, and foods high in impregnated and trans fats.

4. Regular physical exertion can help you maintain a healthy weight, ameliorate your mood, and reduce your threat for habitual conditions. Aim for at least 30 twinkles of moderate- intensity exercise most days of the week.

5. Neglecting your internal health As we progress, it's important to take care of our internal health as well as our physical health. Depression, anxiety, and other internal health conditions can have a negative impact on quality of life.However, seek help from a healthcare professional, If you are passing symptoms of internal illness.

6. Lack of sleep Acceptable sleep is essential for good health. Poor sleep can increase your threat for rotundity, heart complaint, and other conditions. Aim for 7- 8 hours of sleep per night.

7. Avoiding preventative wireworks Regular wireworks for conditions like cancer, high blood pressure, and diabetes can help decry implicit health problems beforehand, when they are easier to treat. Do not skip your regular check- ups with your healthcare provider.

8. Neglecting dental care Oral health is important for overall health. Encounter and floss daily, and see your dentist for regular check- ups and cleanings.

9. Not wearing sunscreen covers your skin from the sun's dangerous shafts by wearing sunscreen with a minimal SPF of 30. This can reduce your threat for skin cancer and unseasonable aging.

10. Social connections are important for emotional good. Maintain connections with family and musketeers, and find openings to join groups or associations that intrigue you. In conclusion, there are several effects to avoid at age 50- 80 in order to promote good health and good health.
These include smoking, drinking too much alcohol, poor diet, inactivity, neglecting your internal health, lack of sleep, avoiding preventative wireworks, neglecting dental care, not wearing sunscreen, and insulation. By making life changes and seeking help from healthcare professionals when demanded, you can maintain good health as you age.

ABOUT AUTHOR

DR.BEN JAPHETH a practical cerebral and health therapist, who works with the world health association for the once 5 times of successful recording awards for psychology and health comforting. He has contributed heavily to the growth and development toW.H.O